HOW TO SLEEP

BETTER

:Expert tips for a good night rest with home remedies

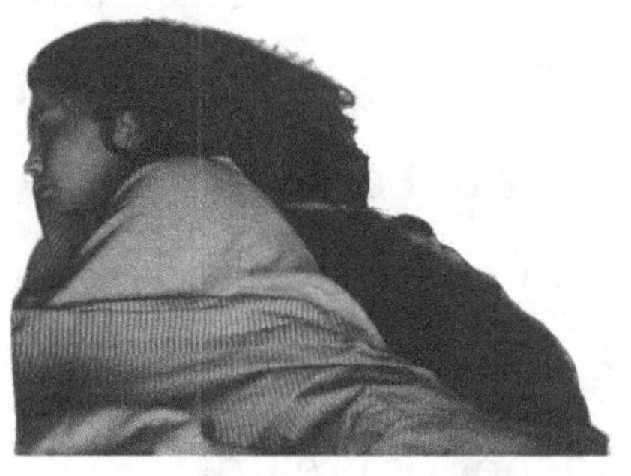

Dr. James E. Davis

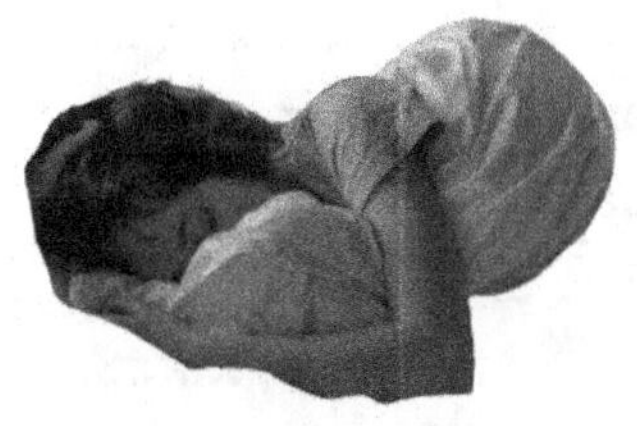

TABLE OF CONTENT

INTRODUCTION

Ensuring a restful night's sleep is essential for your overall well-being. If you find yourself grappling with sleep issues, you may come across a myriad of advice on how to address the problem. However, worry not! We've taken the initiative to delve into the research for you, compiling a comprehensive set of reliable tips to enhance your sleep quality. Our insights draw from the expertise of reputable sources, such as the National Sleep Foundation and Harvard Medical School. These recommendations encompass a spectrum of strategies, ranging from creating a conducive sleep environment to adopting healthy sleep habits.

Rest assured, by incorporating these well-founded tips into your routine, you'll be on your way to enjoying more restful and rejuvenating nights.

Chapter 1: Method 1

Getting to Sleep Quickly (Easy Methods)

Step 1: Initiate your evening relaxation routine by indulging in a soothing warm bath or shower. Beyond its immediate calming effects, this practice induces a subsequent cooling of the body, a crucial element in promoting a more restful sleep. Following this, apply lotion to ensure your skin is not only moisturized but also pleasantly warm.

Step 2: Prior to bedtime, consider incorporating a 400mg magnesium supplement into your routine, ideally consumed 30 to 45 minutes before you plan to sleep. Magnesium is renowned for its role in combating insomnia by reducing the time required to fall asleep, while simultaneously enhancing the overall quality and duration of your sleep. You can easily find magnesium supplements in the vitamin section of your local pharmacy.

Step 3: Embrace the notion of sleeping in the nude, as suggested by sleep specialists at the Cleveland Sleep Clinic. This practice aids in temperature regulation during the night. Achieve an optimal sleeping temperature by layering blankets or a duvet of suitable warmth, accompanied by sheets and pillows. It's advisable to maintain a slightly cooler environment, and if needed, have an extra blanket nearby to ward off potential chills. Pay attention to your extremities, as cold feet can disrupt your sleep. For those who prefer pajamas, opt for loose cotton attire for its breathability.

Step 4: Diversify your sleeping positions to enhance the overall quality of your sleep. Strive for a "mid-line" position, where both your head and neck maintain a straight alignment. Avoid stomach sleeping, as it can be challenging to sustain the proper position and may lead to discomfort. If stomach sleeping is your preference, consider placing the pillow under your hips rather than your head.

Step 5: Select an appropriate pillow to avoid discomfort during sleep. Ensure it's neither too thin nor stacked at an angle, preventing your head from tilting backward uncomfortably. Experiment with placing a pillow between your legs if you sleep on your side, providing support to your hips. Similarly, if you sleep on your back, consider placing a pillow under your legs for added comfort.

Step 6: Diminish your exposure to light an hour or two before bedtime to align with your body's natural circadian rhythm. Bright light before sleep can disrupt your internal clock, signaling confusion between sleep and wakefulness.

Take practical steps such as turning off unnecessary lights, avoiding electronic devices at least two hours before bedtime, and utilizing screen filters like f.lux or Redshift. Eliminate all sources of light in your bedroom, including windows, LED clocks, and other devices.

Step 7: Integrate calming sounds into your sleep environment to enhance relaxation. Utilize a white noise generator featuring soothing sounds like surf, wind, or steam, which lack distinct patterns and aid in redirecting your mind. White noise has demonstrated efficacy not only in expediting the sleep onset but also in masking potential disruptive noises during the night. If white noise machines are unavailable, alternatives such as a fan or a radio tuned between stations to produce static can be equally soothing. Opt for repetitive or ambient music with stable dynamics for a serene pre-sleep ambiance, ensuring it concludes within an hour to avoid disrupting deep sleep.

Additionally, minimize disturbances by turning off or setting your phone to silent mode, particularly if it serves as an alarm. By proactively managing your sleep environment through these steps, you're likely to experience more profound and undisturbed sleep.

EXPERT TIP

I suggest considering the use of wireless sleep headphones when sleeping in a noisy environment. These headphones are designed like a headband, with integrated speakers around the ears, effectively functioning as headphones. Simply ensure that your phone or another compatible device supports Bluetooth, and you can effortlessly and comfortably block out any ambient noise by playing your preferred music or white noise through the headphones. This provides a personalized and soothing auditory environment, promoting a more peaceful and restful night's sleep.

Chapter 2: Method 2

Moderating Your Diet

1. Ensure you have your dinner at least three hours before bedtime. A full stomach can disrupt your sleep, and the heavier the meal, the longer it takes for your stomach to settle. Steer clear of greasy foods, not only because they are unhealthy but also because they can hinder your ability to sleep. Similarly, avoid spicy foods, especially if you've noticed discomfort after consuming them, as they might lead to a stomachache at night.

2. Strike a balance and avoid extremes when it comes to your bedtime hunger. Going to bed on an empty stomach can be as disruptive to your sleep as going to bed with a full stomach. If your stomach is grumbling, consider having a light snack about an hour before bedtime. Opt for snacks that are not high in carbohydrates or sugar. Foods rich in protein, such as turkey, yogurt, soybeans, tuna, and peanuts, containing tryptophan, can help your body produce serotonin, promoting relaxation, and the natural, complex fats can help satiate your hunger.

3. Steer clear of caffeine in the afternoon and evening. This includes coffee, black tea, cocoa, and caffeinated soda.

Even if consumed earlier in the day, caffeine can keep you awake, with its effects lasting up to 12 hours. This caution extends to other stimulants found in energy drinks, regardless of caffeine content. Additionally, avoid tobacco or nicotine products in the evenings.

4. Indulge in a relaxing warm beverage before bedtime. Highly recommended options include a warm glass of milk or chamomile tea. Most herbal teas are suitable, provided they are caffeine-free. However, avoid drinking excessive amounts of fluid right before bedtime.

5. Manage your fluid intake strategically. Refrain from drinking water or other fluids within 1 ½ to 2 hours of your designated bedtime. It's essential to stay adequately hydrated during the day, aiming for at least two liters of water. While a well-hydrated body won't wake you from thirst, consuming a large glass of water just before bed might prompt inconvenient bathroom trips during the night.

6. Exercise caution with alcohol consumption before bed. Although alcohol may induce drowsiness, it can compromise the quality of your sleep as your body processes the alcohol and sugars. Alcohol tends to result in fragmented, shallow sleep,

even if you aren't consciously aware of waking up during the night, ultimately diminishing the restorative benefits of sleep.

Chapter 3: Method 3

Making Your Bed and Bedroom Welcoming

1. Establish a distinct and exclusive purpose for your bedroom, designating it primarily for activities related to bedtime and relaxation. The intention is to create a consistent association between the bedroom and rest, facilitating a seamless transition into sleep. Discourage the engagement in stress-inducing activities, such as work or computer usage, within the bedroom confines. Instead, channel the focus towards tranquil pursuits like reading, partaking in relaxing projects, or sharing intimate moments with a partner.

Reinforce the notion of the bed being solely reserved for sleep, emphasizing its role as an exclusive sanctuary for restorative rest.

2. Elevate the comfort quotient of your bedroom to transform it into a haven that is inherently conducive to restful sleep. The principle is grounded in the belief that a more inviting and comfortable bed, as well as the surrounding environment, fosters an atmosphere conducive to tranquil sleep. Enforce darkness within your sleeping space to minimize external disturbances and amplify the overall sensory environment that promotes rest.

3. Cultivate a positive emotional connection with your room through a commitment to cleanliness and organizational order. Regular cleaning rituals, encompassing tasks such as dusting, vacuuming, and decluttering, contribute not only to an overall sense of well-being but also help mitigate potential disruptors like allergies. The act of maintaining a clean bed, accomplished through the regular washing of sheets and pillowcases, further bolsters the conducive nature of the sleep environment.

4. Invest concerted efforts into enhancing the aesthetics of your room to positively influence your overall mood. Simple adjustments,

whether in the form of updating bedding or refreshing wall paint, can subtly and gradually impact the ambiance. Incorporating blackout drapes, shades, or blinds to manage light levels and strategically considering temperature regulation tactics further optimize the sleep-inducing conditions.

5. Prioritize the diligent care of your mattress, recognizing signs for potential replacement after five to seven years of consistent use. Be attuned to indicators such as feeling springs or ridges beneath the surface or experiencing excessive movement during sleep. Concurrently, explore the concept of assessing your sleep quality in different beds,

an approach that can serve as a valuable guide in determining the opportune moment to invest in a new mattress.

6. Delve into the realm of possibilities surrounding a new mattress, with a specific focus on options tailored to individual preferences and needs. Adjustable mattresses, allowing for personalized firmness for both partners, present an attractive solution for accommodating varied comfort requirements. Equally noteworthy are memory foam mattresses, characterized by their adaptive nature, conforming to body contours as they warm up.

This feature proves particularly beneficial for addressing pressure points and catering to the specific needs of individuals with joint concerns. The exploration of these alternatives is poised to contribute not only to an enhanced sleep experience but also to an overarching sense of holistic well-being.

Chapter 4: Method 4

Changing Your Daily Routine

1. Cultivate a consistent sleep routine by adhering to the same bedtime and wake-up time every day. Deviating from these times by more than an hour can significantly disrupt your sleep quality by interfering with your circadian rhythm, the internal biological clock that regulates various bodily functions, including sleep-wake cycles.

Maintain this regular sleep schedule, even during weekends, to reinforce your body's natural rhythm. Even on occasions when you may need to retire to bed later than usual, strive to wake up at your customary time to maintain the stability of your sleep pattern.

Commit to immediate action upon the sounding of your alarm clock each morning. Resist the temptation to linger in bed or succumb to the allure of the snooze button. Establishing a habit of getting up promptly contributes to the consistency of your sleep-wake routine, enhancing overall sleep quality and reinforcing a healthy circadian rhythm.

EXPERT TIP

1. Implementing a consistent bedtime routine can be effortlessly achieved by setting an alarm to mark the commencement of winding down activities. This pre-sleep routine includes essential tasks like changing into pajamas, engaging in dental hygiene, and generally preparing for a restful night's sleep. By adhering to this structured routine, you signal to your body that it's time to transition into a state conducive to sleep.

2. Tailoring your sleep duration to meet your individual needs is paramount. Acknowledge that people require varying amounts of sleep, and if you find yourself taking more than 30 minutes to

fall asleep or experiencing prolonged wakefulness during the night, consider adjusting your sleep time. Gradual reductions, in 15-minute intervals each week, can lead to a more optimized sleep duration. Embrace initial fatigue as your body adapts, striving for a balance that ensures deep, continuous sleep without unnecessary excess.

3. The establishment of a consistent sleep routine involves engaging in the same pre-sleep activities each night. For an evening characterized by tranquility, consider incorporating ambient music, soft candlelight, and deliberate breathing exercises or meditation to relax both your body and mind.

The gradual dimming of your environment as you transition to the bedroom further enhances the soothing quality of this pre-sleep routine.

4. Deep breathing relaxation techniques, performed before bedtime, can contribute to cultivating a calm mental and physical state. Find a comfortable, minimally lit space, introduce calming music, and take a few moments to clear your mind. Inhale positive imagery, focusing on your breath to induce relaxation. Maintaining this practice for 10 minutes nightly, supplemented by the addition of lavender oil to your pillow, can enhance the overall calming effects.

5. Integrate regular exercise into your daily routine to promote a deeper and more restful sleep. Recognize that physical exertion aids the body's recovery process during sleep. Engage in activities such as running, swimming, or regular exercise to contribute to a more robust sleep cycle. To allow your body to naturally wind down, avoid exercising within 2 hours of bedtime.

6. Strategically consider the benefits of short naps during the day to combat daytime drowsiness. If your schedule permits, indulge in a brief 15-minute nap when needed, setting a timer to prevent oversleeping. This approach allows for a quick refreshment without the potential grogginess associated with

more extended periods of daytime sleep. By incorporating these practices into your routine, you can foster improved sleep quality and overall well-being.

Chapter 5: Method 5

Using Medication for Better Sleep

1. Explore the use of melatonin as a potential aid for sleep. Melatonin, a hormone produced by the pineal gland in the brain, plays a crucial role in regulating sleep-wake cycles.

The pineal gland actively converts serotonin to melatonin in the absence of light, promoting a sense of drowsiness. Consulting with your physician before incorporating melatonin supplements is crucial, as it is a hormone, similar to estrogen or testosterone. While melatonin is considered a natural sleep inducer, its use should be approached with caution, and professional guidance is advisable.

2.   Consider plain antihistamine products with sedative effects as a temporary solution for inducing drowsiness. Ensure that the product chosen does not contain additional ingredients such as pain relievers, decongestants, or expectorants. Use these products sparingly, limiting their use to a night or two, as tolerance can develop quickly. Carefully read the labels and start with half or less of the recommended dose to avoid potential side effects. It is advisable to be in a lying position in bed when the drowsiness sets in.

If you are using prescription medications, consult with your doctor before introducing any additional substances, as unintended interactions could have adverse effects. It is essential to strictly adhere to prescribed dosages and recommended durations to prevent misuse or dependency on sedatives.

3. Communicate any concerns about potential sleep disorders to your doctor. Common sleep disorders such as insomnia, narcolepsy, and parasomnias can significantly impact sleep quality. If diagnosed with any of these conditions, your doctor can recommend appropriate treatment strategies. Additionally, conditions like anxiety, depression, premenstrual syndrome (PMS),

and certain medications may contribute to sleep difficulties and should be addressed through consultation with a healthcare professional. Proactively discussing your sleep concerns with your doctor allows for a comprehensive evaluation and tailored interventions to improve overall sleep health.

Question

Does my food have an impact on how well I sleep during the night?
Certain dietary choices can impact your comfort when falling asleep. Notably, substances like alcohol, caffeine, and monosodium glutamate (MSG) can potentially disrupt your sleep.

It's advisable to avoid consuming these substances, as well as large meals, close to bedtime to promote a more comfortable and restful sleep experience.

1. Alcohol: While alcohol might induce drowsiness, it can lead to disrupted sleep patterns, causing more shallow and fragmented sleep. It's recommended to limit alcohol intake, especially in the hours leading up to bedtime.

2. Caffeine: Found in coffee, tea, chocolate, and some sodas, caffeine is a stimulant that can interfere with the ability to fall asleep. It's prudent to avoid caffeinated beverages and foods, particularly in the hours preceding bedtime.

3. MSG (Monosodium Glutamate): MSG, commonly used as a flavor enhancer in many processed foods, may cause discomfort in some individuals. It's wise to be mindful of MSG-containing foods, especially in the evening, to prevent potential disruptions to your sleep.

4. Large Meals: Consuming substantial meals close to bedtime can lead to discomfort, indigestion, and potential sleep disturbances. Opt for lighter, easily digestible snacks if you feel the need to eat before bedtime.

By being mindful of your dietary choices and avoiding these substances and large meals before bedtime, you can contribute to a more conducive environment for falling asleep and enjoying a restful night.

Tips

1. Incorporate Daily Probiotics for Improved Sleep: Including probiotics in your daily routine has shown positive effects on sleep. Probiotics, which promote a healthy balance of gut bacteria, may influence various bodily functions, including those related to sleep regulation.

Consider integrating probiotic-rich foods like yogurt, kefir, sauerkraut, or taking a daily probiotic supplement to potentially enhance your sleep quality.

2. Establish a Pre-Bedtime Bathroom Routine: Always ensure to visit the restroom before heading to bed. This simple yet effective practice can help

minimize disruptions during the night, allowing for a more uninterrupted and restful sleep. Reducing the likelihood of waking up to use the bathroom contributes to a smoother sleep cycle.

3. Engage in Bedtime Reading: Reading a book before bedtime is a time-honored and relaxing ritual that can promote better sleep. Opt for a physical book or an e-reader with a warm light setting to avoid the stimulating effects of bright screens. Reading can help shift your focus away from daily stressors and electronic devices, creating a conducive mental environment for winding down and preparing for a good night's sleep.

1. Avoid Falling Asleep with the TV On: Steer clear of falling asleep with the television on, as it can condition your body to rely on background noise for sleep. This dependency on noise may make it challenging to fall asleep in a quiet environment, especially if you wake up during the night. Cultivate a sleep-friendly environment by minimizing reliance on external stimuli.

2. Exercise Caution with Chamomile Tea: If you have a ragweed allergy or are taking blood thinners, exercise caution when considering chamomile tea as a sleep aid. While chamomile is a popular choice for its calming properties, it's essential to be aware of potential interactions or allergic reactions based on individual health considerations.

3. Mind Fire Safety When Covering Light Sources: If you choose to cover sources of light in your bedroom for better sleep, prioritize safety to avoid fire hazards. Avoid covering heat-emitting sources like light bulbs with combustible materials. When using candles, ensure they are extinguished before sleep and never leave them unattended. If there's uncertainty about staying awake to blow out candles, consider alternative lighting options or use them cautiously.

4. Exercise Caution with Sleep Medication: Keep a vigilant eye on your use of sleep medication, whether over-the-counter or prescription, as dependence can develop. Continuous reliance on such medications may hinder your ability to fall asleep naturally. Additionally, be aware of potential side effects that could impact your daily routine and diminish overall sleep quality. Regularly assess the necessity and impact of sleep aids on your sleep health.

Chapter 6: Bonus

20 easy and quick home remedies for better sleep

1. Chamomile Tea:

- Drink a cup of chamomile tea before bedtime to relax your mind and body.

2. Warm Milk with Honey:

- Warm milk contains tryptophan, a natural sleep inducer, and honey helps regulate blood sugar levels.

3. Lavender Essential Oil:

- Place a few drops of lavender essential oil on your pillow or use a diffuser to promote relaxation.

4. Valerian Root Tea:

- Valerian root has sedative properties; try drinking valerian tea before bedtime.

5. Banana Tea:

- Boil a banana (with the peel) to make a soothing tea that contains sleep-promoting nutrients.

6. Magnesium-Rich Foods:

- Consume magnesium-rich foods like nuts, seeds, and dark chocolate, as magnesium helps regulate sleep.

7. Aromatherapy with Bergamot:

- Inhale the aroma of bergamot essential oil to reduce anxiety and promote relaxation.

8. Limit Caffeine Intake:

- Avoid caffeine-containing beverages in the evening, as they can interfere with sleep.

9. Create a Bedtime Routine:

- Create a consistent bedtime routine to alert your body that it's time to wind down.

10. Herbal Sleep Pillow:

- Fill a small pillow with herbs like lavender, chamomile, and mint to place under your regular pillow.

11. Yoga and Stretching:

- Engage in gentle yoga or stretching exercises to relax your muscles and ease tension.

12. Dark Room Environment:

- Ensure your bedroom is completely dark, as exposure to light can disrupt your circadian rhythm.

13. White Noise Machine:

- Use a white noise machine or app to drown out background noises that may disturb your sleep.

14. Limit Electronic Devices:

- Avoid electronic devices before bedtime, as the blue light emitted can interfere with melatonin production.

15. Warm Bath with Epsom Salt:

- Take a warm bath with Epsom salt to relax muscles and promote a sense of calm.

16. Ginger Tea:

- Ginger tea can help with digestion, preventing discomfort that may disturb your sleep.

17. Herbal Sleep Elixir:

- Mix passionflower and lemon balm extracts in warm water for a calming herbal sleep elixir.

18. Acupressure:

- Try acupressure techniques, focusing on points like the base of your skull and the inner wrist.

19. Tart Cherry Juice:

- Tart cherry juice is a natural source of melatonin; consider drinking a small amount before bedtime.

20. Deep Breathing Exercises:

- Perform some deep breathing exercises to calm your nerves and promote relaxation.

CONCLUSION

Enhancing your sleep quality can be achieved through simple adjustments to your sleep environment and daily routine. Consider incorporating the following practices for improved rest:

1. Optimal Sleeping Temperature: Improve your sleep environment by keeping your bedroom cool. The brain associates lower temperatures with bedtime, and sleeping in a colder room can enhance your overall sleep quality. Maintain a comfortable and cool atmosphere to promote restful sleep.

2. Minimize Screen Time Before Bed: Reduce exposure to screens, such as phones, tablets, and computers, at least two hours before bedtime. If screen use is unavoidable, activate nighttime mode to mitigate the impact of blue light, which can interfere with your body's natural sleep-wake cycle. Minimizing screen time before bed helps signal to your brain that it's time to wind down.

3. Utilize White Noise with a Fan: Employ a fan in your bedroom to create white noise, fostering a calming environment conducive to relaxation. The gentle hum of a fan can drown out background noises, helping your mind unwind as you transition into sleep. This auditory backdrop can contribute to a more serene and peaceful sleeping environment.

4. Establish Consistent Sleep Patterns: Strive to maintain a consistent sleep schedule by going to bed and waking up at the same time every day. This practice helps regulate your circadian rhythm, aligning your body's internal clock with a predictable sleep-wake cycle. Consistency in sleep patterns allows your body to optimize the restorative benefits of sleep over the long term.